I0407208

52

INSPIRATIONS

FOR HEALTHY

Nutrition

DEDICATION

I would like to dedicate this book to my wife for her loving being that harmonizes with my dreams and realities.

I would also like to convey the immense gratitude I have for my family and friends as they are my ultimate treasures.

INTRODUCTION

This simple book is designed to help you take simple steps toward healthier nutrition.

I hope you will find that it is a soft and fun way to embrace better nutrition over your year. Like a fortune cookie, this book is meant to be easy and enjoyable - filled with simple exercises to help you live a healthy life.

Through the journey of self-love I have found the ability to give love, receive love, and create a loving space around myself. I want to help you do that too. I'm so glad you've picked up this book and you're taking these small actions for yourself and for those you love. One last thing, I've left blank space throughout the book to the left of every inspiration for you to add notes and thoughts from your conversations.

Good luck and have fun!

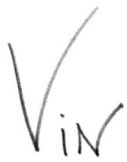

Accept who you are and where you are, this is your starting point

Drink one extra glass of water today

Eat one fruit or vegetable today anyway you like

Start your day with a hot honey lemon water

Walk slowly through the produce aisle two times this week

Create time and space in your life for eating

Try meditating for 1 minute.

Helpful Tip
Simply close your eyes, be silent and focus on your breathing

Start to look for nutritional value in your food

Observe everything you want to eat today, just start by paying attention

Cut artificial sweeteners and use natural alternatives like real honey and maple syrup

Find a healthy source of good news

Resources
Find a list of our favorites in the resources
section at the back of the book

Look for new combinations of food that are healthier where you already eat

Forgo one alcoholic beverage or one dessert this week

Collect a new idea or recipe that you would like to try

Make a list of 5 reasons why you're eating healthier

Bonus Points
Use our template in our resources and put it somewhere you can see every day

Slow down while you are eating

Take time for chewing, talking,
thinking and breathing.

Fill your plate with colors today for lunch

Add a variety of colors with your starches, vegetables and fruits

Seek out foods that are made from scratch

Generally looking to cut out mass produced foods, stabilizers and preservatives.

Think about how much water is in the food you eat

Helpful Tip
Eat more foods with high water content!

Clean out the salad dressings

Healthy Tip
Remove the dressings with high fat,
high sugar or high calories.

Put some almond butter on a carrot or celery stick for a snack

Make a list of foods that make you feel strong and healthy

Now make a list of foods that make you feel weak & unhealthy

Make a Plan
Reduce your frequency around these foods
and plan how you will resist these foods

Have a spa day

Healthy Tip
Treat yourself to a stress relieving day and
work on creating a regular self-care practice

Focus on something beautiful three times today

Move your legs 30 minutes today

Bonus Points
Arrange for a standing desk or workplace and don't stay seated all day. Let's burn some calories while we're on the clock!

Take time to appreciate your meal

Think About It
Reflect on the amazing world your food comes through and the people, plants, animals and everything that makes it all possible.

Clean out the fridge throw the bad habits and old things away

Track your treats and alcohol

Healthy Tip
Know exactly how many you are consuming
and try spacing them out with healthy
alternatives in between.

Get a rice steamer to make your own rice

Bonus Points
Put your veggies on top of the veggie
steaming tray for added nutrition!

Try watering down your fruit juices to add more hydration and less sugar

Eat fruits on an empty stomach as they are very quick to digest

Resources
Check out our *10 Tips for Food Sequencing*
at the back of the book

Drink a second glass of water today

Eat a second raw fruit or vegetable that you prepare today

Enjoy audio that calms and soothes you around meals

Free Resources
Check our resources for a downloadable
audio tracks created by Vin

Find or create a peaceful sign for your kitchen

Free Resources
Check our resources for an example

Buy a new knife or get your knives sharpened at the hardware store

Cut out one bleached or refined food item

Examples
White bread, saltines, crackers, cereal.

Replace high fructose corn syrup with natural sugar or all natural products

Take a deep breath and smile three times today

Buy yourself a cooler to bring leftovers, fruits and vegetables along with you during your day

Cut your pizza slices in half

Super Smart!
This doubles the amount of slices in a pie and gives you and your family half-slice options.

Remember good sources of proteins, fats and carbs

Proteins: meat, beans, nuts, fish and eggs.
Fats: meats, nuts, fish, eggs, avocados.
Carbs: veggies, yams, potatoes, rice, roots.

Find someone who shares your interests and goals

You can each benefit from sharing experiences and supporting each other.

Clean out your cabinets

Give away or throw away foods that don't meet your health goals and make a commitment to stop buying them

Use olive oil & smart balance spreads to cut down on butter

Buy yourself a new mug for herbal tea and try at night or after a meal

Eat vegetables first before you enjoy a starch and protein in your next meal

Keep to your shopping list

Resources
Check out our *10 Tips for Meal Planning*
at the back of the book

Look for healthy
alternatives to
the vending
machine snacks
(like apples)

Visit your local farmers market and pick something up off the shelf

Give yourself a reward for eating better!

RESOURCES

#11 Good News

Here are some of our favorite sources of good news. These include websites with articles, books and more!

Free Daily Positive News
theoptimist.com

Greater Good Center at Berkeley
greatergood.berkeley.edu

***Abundance* by Peter Diamandis**
abundancethebook.com

The Institute for Global Happiness
globalhappiness.org/resources

Daily Positive Awesome Things
1000awesomethings.com

Ways to Happier World
actionforhappiness.org

#15 Your Reasons

Your 5 reasons why you're eating healthier

#1

_____

#2

_____

#3

_____

#4

_____

#5

_____

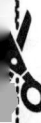

#32 Food Sequencing
Our *Tips for Food Sequencing*

Burps, farts and heartburn are the worst, but where do they come from? While experiencing some gas in the digestive track is normal much of it can be avoided by using food sequencing.

Food sequencing is paying attention to what's in your stomach and what you're about to eat and knowing how those foods interact together. Below are our *10 Tips for Food Sequencing* and on the next page a *Simple Guide to Food Digestion Times.*

10 Tips for Food Sequencing
1. Eat fruit first so it doesn't sit on other food and ferment in the digestive track.
2. Know that fruits digest quickest, often in 25 minutes or shorter.
3. Know that vegetables digest quicker than proteins (beans and nuts, then meats).
4. Eat "hard to digest foods" last in meals.
5. Give time for digestion between meals and snacks.
6. Consume water during off-peak digestion times.
7. Start breakfast with a fruit plate.
8. Then proceed to a protein & starch portion.
9. For lunch have a large salad and finish with a protein/carbohydrate portion.
10. For dinner start with a vegetable plate and then proceed to a protein & starch portion.

Simple Guide to Food Digestion Times

Fruits

Generally digests very quickly 10-25 minutes	First thing in the morning or anytime stomach is empty	May ferment when left to sit too long waiting for other foods to digest

Vegetables

Generally digests 30-60 minutes	Vegetables eaten first during a meal helps consuming 6 portions	Getting used to eating vegetables gradually increasing portions

Nuts & Seeds

Generally 1-2 hours	Can be a great source of protein and calories	Plan to consume more liquids

Meats

Generally 2+ hours	Raw meats take longer to digest	Turkey is an easier meat to digest

#32 Relaxing Music

To download free tracks of wonderful relaxing music, please visit www.bodybybari.com/music

There you can find amazing tracks designed by Vin Ramirez to help you relax, slow down and enjoy your meals even more.

These include tracks of space-enhancing music as well as meditations and affirmations.

#36 Peaceful Sign

On the next page you will find a peaceful sign designed by Vin Ramirez that you can cut out of the book or just use to inspire you.

Smile

Laugh

Play

Music revel in it Easy Loose

Gratitude

Thank you for my connection to all energies past present & future, for my emotions acting as a guidance to align with my true intentions
Music

Praise Bless Joy
Appreciate

Harmony

Joy Flowing unfolding

Delightful
Music
Giving

Allow Freedom
volunteer

Abundance

Going with the flow of my energy

Praise Always Music Forgiveness

Brotherly love Breathe Selflove World Love

Being & Let Being

#49 Meal Planning

Our 10 Tips for Meal Planning

1. Acknowledge the time and space it takes to plan your meals and give yourself the permission to take that time for yourself.
2. Explore many resources to discover what type of meal planning suits your lifestyle. Browse the internet and magazines, and talk with friends and social networks to find what works for you.
3. Discover the favorite recipes of your partner, family & friends and collect them.
4. Think about what days of the week feel best for shopping and what days feel best for cooking.
5. Consider healthy resources such as healthy pre-prepared at your local market to aid in meal preparations.
6. If you enjoy buying things that are seasonal and on sale, try freezing them in large batches. This makes it easy for you to pull out meal-sized portions from the freezer.
7. Choose food recipes that you will enjoy preparing, enjoy eating as leftovers and can be frozen easily.
8. Don't overload your freezer, have a plan for when you'll use it and keep everything well-labeled.
9. In cabinets make sure you can see everything and if the expiration dates has passed, throw it out.
10. Don't overstock, remember: clean it out, cook it up, freeze it or throw it out.

#49 Shopping List
A Simple List to Bring Shopping

It's Always A Good Idea to Buy:

○ Fruit #1 (as many as you like)
○ Fruit #2 (as many as you like)
○ Fruit #3 (as many as you like)
○ A dark leafy green vegetable and broccoli
○ Earthy Vegetable #1 (as many as you like)
○ Colorful vegetable #1 (as many as you like)
○ Colorful vegetable #2 (as many as you like)
○ Rices and grains
○ Low-fat meats
○ Herbal teas

Great Fruits
Apples, oranges, watermelons, bananas, grapes, pineapples, grapefruit, mangos, peaches, kiwi, strawberries and cantaloupe.

Great Earthy Vegetables
Onions, garlic, mushrooms, leeks, scallions, shallots, and ginger.

Great Colorful Vegetables
Peppers, sweet potatoes, carrots, squash, beets, tomatoes, green beans, and cucumbers.

ABOUT THE AUTHOR

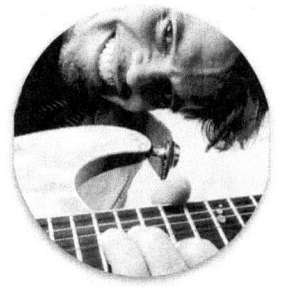

Vincent Ramirez is a graduate of Culinary Institute of America and has over three decades of experience as a professional chef and nutrition expert.

Currently Vin lives in Woodstock, Vermont with his wonderful wife where he enjoys an artist lifestyle. He creates relaxation therapy, audio and video exercises and mindfulness resources which you can find at BodybyBari.com.

52 Inspirations for Healthy Nutrition is his first book.

ABOUT THE EDITOR

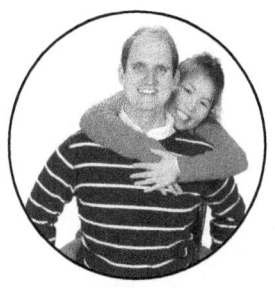

Travis Hellstrom is a leadership coach, professor and author who loves helping people lead happy and simple lives.

He also loves writing books and sharing them with the world with incredible friends like Vin and Bari. He counts himself lucky to be one of the many people inspired by their love, optimism and creativity.

Travis is the author of the *Peace Corps Volunteer's Handbook*, *The Dalai Lama Book of Quotes*, *52 Inspirations for Healthy Loving Couples, 52 Questions for a Better Relationship* and several other books.

To find them and read more from Travis visit: TravisHellstrom.com.